PREDIABETES

FOOD LIST

INTRODUCTION

The Prediabetes Food List

In a world where dietary choices are crucial to our health, "The Prediabetes Food List" stands out as an essential guide for those looking to take charge of their health journey. This meticulously researched book offers comprehensive insights specifically for individuals at the critical stage of prediabetes.

As prediabetes becomes increasingly common worldwide, understanding dietary intervention is crucial. This book goes beyond a basic list of foods; it serves as a beacon of empowerment and sustainable change. It provides a wealth of knowledge, not just about which foods to include or avoid, but also about the scientific principles behind these choices, effective meal planning strategies, and lifestyle adjustments that can profoundly influence your prediabetic journey.

Whether you are proactively trying to prevent diabetes or have recently been diagnosed with prediabetes, this guide is here to help. It transforms the idea of a food list into a powerful tool for developing mindful eating habits, making informed choices, and charting a course toward a healthier future. The "Prediabetes Food List" is more than a book; it is a vital companion on your journey to reclaim your health and embrace a life of vitality.

TABLE OF CONTENT

RECIPES

RECIPES

GREEK SALAD WITH GRILLED CHICKEN OR SHRIMP

A Greek salad with grilled chicken or shrimp is a great option for those with prediabetes because it features a low glycemic index and is packed with nutrients. This tasty and filling dish combines crisp vegetables like cucumbers, tomatoes, and red onions with tangy Kalamata olives, creamy feta cheese, and a light olive oil and lemon juice dressing. Adding lean, protein-rich grilled chicken or shrimp makes it a balanced meal choice for managing blood sugar levels.

The main advantage of Greek salad for prediabetes is its low glycemic index. The glycemic index (GI) measures how foods affect blood sugar levels. High GI foods can cause quick spikes in blood sugar, which is problematic for people with prediabetes. Since Greek salad is mostly made up of vegetables, which have a low GI, the carbohydrates in the salad are digested slowly, leading to a gradual release of glucose and preventing significant blood sugar spikes.

Moreover, Greek salad is rich in essential nutrients. Vegetables like cucumbers offer vitamins C and K and are hydrating, while tomatoes are high in lycopene, an antioxidant linked to a lower risk of chronic diseases. Kalamata olives provide heart-healthy monounsaturated fats, and feta cheese adds calcium and protein. The grilled chicken or shrimp contributes lean protein, important for muscle health and satiety.

Making Greek salad with grilled chicken or shrimp is straightforward. Start by grilling the protein until it's fully cooked and slightly charred for added flavor. Meanwhile, chop the cucumbers, tomatoes, and red onions into bite-sized pieces. Mix these vegetables with Kalamata olives and crumbled feta cheese in a large bowl. In a separate small bowl, whisk together olive oil, lemon juice, salt, and pepper to make the dressing. Pour the dressing over the salad and toss gently to coat everything evenly. Finally, top with the grilled chicken or shrimp, and the salad is ready to serve. This Mediterranean-inspired dish is both nutritious and satisfying, supporting blood sugar control for those with prediabetes.

VEGGIE AND BEAN BURRITO BOWL WITH BROWN RICE AND SALSA

A veggie and bean burrito bowl with brown rice and salsa is a flavorful and nutritious choice for individuals with prediabetes. This filling meal offers several benefits for blood sugar management and overall health.

Brown rice, the base of this dish, is a complex carbohydrate with a low glycemic index, resulting in a gradual impact on blood sugar compared to white rice. It's also high in fiber, which aids digestion and helps control blood sugar levels, and is rich in essential nutrients like magnesium and B vitamins, beneficial for those with prediabetes.

The vegetable and bean components of the burrito bowl are nutrient-dense without added sugars or refined carbs. Vegetables such as bell peppers, onions, and tomatoes are full of vitamins, minerals, and fiber. Beans like black or pinto beans provide plant-based protein and fiber, which help regulate blood sugar.

To make this dish, start by cooking the brown rice according to the package directions. While the rice is cooking, sauté a mix of bell peppers, onions, and any additional vegetables in a bit of olive oil until they are tender. Add the beans and heat them through, seasoning with spices like cumin, paprika, and chili powder for extra flavor.

Once everything is cooked, assemble your burrito bowl with a base of brown rice. Top it with the vegetable and bean mixture. Add a spoonful of salsa or homemade tomato salsa for extra zest and freshness. For additional garnish, consider adding fresh cilantro, avocado slices, or a squeeze of lime.

This veggie and bean burrito bowl with brown rice and salsa offers a satisfying and delicious meal for those managing prediabetes, thanks to its low-glycemic index ingredients. The combination of whole grains, vegetables, and legumes provides a well-balanced, nutrient-rich dish that is both diabetes-friendly and flavorful.

To prepare a similar meal, you can marinate shrimp in a mixture of olive oil, lemon juice, garlic, and herbs. While the shrimp marinates for 20-30 minutes, prepare a side salad with mixed greens, cherry tomatoes, cucumber slices, and bell peppers. Cook whole grain couscous according to the package instructions. After marinating, thread the shrimp onto skewers and grill them for a few minutes on each side until they turn pink and opaque. Serve the grilled shrimp skewers with the side salad and couscous for a complete, satisfying meal that supports stable blood sugar levels and overall health.

GRILLED SHRIMP SKEWERS WITH A SIDE SALAD AND WHOLE GRAIN COUSCOUS

Grilled shrimp skewers with a side salad and whole grain couscous is a nutritious and tasty option for those with prediabetes. Shrimp offers a low-calorie, lean protein source enriched with omega-3 fatty acids, which can enhance insulin sensitivity and decrease inflammation. It also provides essential vitamins and minerals, including vitamin B12, selenium, and zinc, which support heart health and help regulate blood sugar.

Adding a side salad boosts the meal's nutritional profile with high fiber and a variety of vegetables like leafy greens, tomatoes, cucumbers, and bell peppers. These ingredients are low in calories but packed with vitamins, minerals, and antioxidants, which help manage blood sugar, promote satiety, and prevent complications associated with prediabetes.

Whole grain couscous complements the dish with its complex carbohydrates, fiber, and essential nutrients like magnesium and phosphorus. These components help slow digestion and avoid rapid blood sugar spikes. The fiber content in couscous also supports weight management by increasing feelings of fullness and lowering overall calorie consumption.

BLACK BEAN AND VEGETABLE ENCHILADAS WITH A SIDE OF SALSA AND BROWN RICE

Black bean and vegetable enchiladas with a side of salsa and brown rice make a nutritious and satisfying choice for those with prediabetes. This dish is not only delicious but also supports blood sugar management and overall health.

Black beans are a fantastic option for individuals with prediabetes, offering a combination of protein, fiber, and complex carbohydrates. These components help slow digestion and the release of glucose into the bloodstream, preventing sudden spikes in blood sugar. The complex carbohydrates in black beans provide a steady release of energy, avoiding rapid fluctuations in blood sugar levels.

Adding a variety of vegetables to the enchiladas boosts their nutritional value while keeping the meal low in calories and carbohydrates. Vegetables like bell peppers, onions, zucchini, and spinach offer a range of vitamins, minerals, and antioxidants that contribute to overall health. They also increase the fiber content of the dish, which aids digestion, enhances satiety, and supports weight management.

To prepare the enchiladas, begin by sautéing the vegetables in a bit of olive oil until tender. Mix in the black beans and season with cumin, paprika, and chili powder for extra flavor. Spoon the filling onto corn tortillas, roll them up, and place them in a baking dish. Top with a homemade salsa made from diced tomatoes, onions, cilantro, lime juice, and a hint of jalapeño for a zesty touch. Bake until the tortillas are crispy and the flavors have melded together. Serve the enchiladas with a portion of nutty brown rice for a complete and balanced meal.

Black bean and vegetable enchiladas with salsa and brown rice offer a diabetes-friendly, nutritious meal. The combination of protein, fiber, and complex carbohydrates in the black beans, along with the nutrient-rich vegetables and low glycemic index of brown rice, helps maintain stable blood sugar levels while delivering a delicious and fulfilling meal.

BAKED TOFU WITH ROASTED SWEET POTATOES AND STEAMED GREEN BEANS

Baked tofu with roasted sweet potatoes and steamed green beans is a flavorful and nutritious meal especially suited for those with prediabetes. Tofu, derived from soybeans, provides a valuable plant-based protein that helps stabilize blood sugar levels and improve insulin sensitivity. It's low in fat and cholesterol, making it heart-healthy for those concerned about diabetes.

Roasted sweet potatoes add a delightful sweetness and are rich in fiber, vitamins, and minerals. Their high fiber content helps manage blood sugar levels by slowing the digestion and absorption of carbohydrates. Additionally, sweet potatoes are packed with beta-carotene, an antioxidant that may lower the risk of diabetes-related complications.

Steamed green beans offer a burst of essential nutrients such as vitamin C, vitamin K, and folate. These nutrients enhance blood circulation, immune function, and overall health. Together, these ingredients create a balanced, low-calorie, and nutrient-dense meal that supports blood sugar management and healthy weight maintenance.

To prepare this meal, preheat your oven to 400°F (200°C). Cut the tofu into cubes and marinate it with a mixture of soy sauce, garlic, and ginger. While the tofu marinates, peel and dice the sweet potatoes into bite-sized pieces. Toss them in olive oil, salt, and optional seasonings like paprika or cinnamon. Arrange the marinated tofu and seasoned sweet potatoes on a baking sheet and roast for about 25-30 minutes until golden and crispy. Steam the green beans for 5-7 minutes until tender yet bright green. Serve the baked tofu over the roasted sweet potatoes, accompanied by the steamed green beans. This vibrant and tasty dish will not only please your palate but also support your health and well-being if you have prediabetes.

SPINACH AND FETA OMELET WITH WHOLE WHEAT TOAST

A spinach and feta omelet with whole wheat toast is a tasty and nutritious meal ideal for individuals with prediabetes. This dish is rich in essential nutrients and low in carbohydrates, making it a great choice for managing blood sugar levels and supporting overall health.

Spinach, the main ingredient, is a leafy green vegetable packed with vitamins A, C, and K, as well as minerals like iron and magnesium. Its low calorie and high fiber content make it excellent for controlling blood sugar levels, as fiber slows carbohydrate digestion and prevents rapid spikes in blood sugar.

Feta cheese enhances the omelet's flavor and adds nutritional value. It provides protein, calcium, and vitamins B6 and B12. Protein helps regulate blood sugar by slowing glucose absorption, while calcium supports bone health and B vitamins aid in nervous system function.

Paired with whole wheat toast, this meal benefits from the toast's higher fiber content compared to refined white bread. Whole wheat bread contains important nutrients such as folate, magnesium, and selenium, which contribute to better digestion and blood sugar control.

To prepare the omelet, whisk eggs with fresh spinach leaves and crumbled feta cheese. Heat a non-stick pan over medium heat, pour in the egg mixture, and cook until the edges start to set. Fold the omelet in half and cook until fully set. Serve with a slice of toasted whole wheat bread for a balanced and satisfying meal.

A spinach and feta omelet with whole wheat toast offers a healthy, low-carb option for managing prediabetes. Its nutrient-rich ingredients and high fiber content help regulate blood sugar levels and provide various health benefits.

QUINOA-STUFFED BELL PEPPERS WITH LEAN GROUND TURKEY OR TOFU

Quinoa-stuffed bell peppers with lean ground turkey or tofu is a healthy and flavorful meal ideal for individuals with prediabetes. This dish combines nutrient-dense ingredients like quinoa, fiber-rich bell peppers, and a choice of lean protein, offering numerous health benefits.

Quinoa is a highly nutritious grain rich in fiber, protein, vitamins, and minerals. Its low glycemic index helps regulate blood sugar levels and prevent spikes, making it a great choice for managing prediabetes. Additionally, quinoa is a good source of magnesium, which supports insulin sensitivity and helps prevent type 2 diabetes.

Bell peppers are packed with antioxidants, vitamins A and C, and fiber. Low in calories and glycemic index, they complement the quinoa perfectly, providing a nutrient-rich, satisfying meal.

Lean ground turkey or tofu can be used as the protein source. Lean ground turkey offers high-quality protein that supports muscle health and weight management while being low in fat. Tofu, a plant-based alternative, is suitable for vegetarians and vegans. It's low in saturated fat and cholesterol, making it heart-healthy and beneficial for blood sugar control.

Preparation Steps:

Preheat the oven and cook quinoa according to package instructions.

Prepare bell peppers by cutting off the tops and removing seeds.

Cook the ground turkey or tofu in a pan with olive oil and seasonings until fully cooked.

Combine the cooked quinoa and protein in a mixing bowl.

Stuff the mixture into the bell peppers and bake until the peppers are tender and the filling is golden brown.

Quinoa-stuffed bell peppers with lean ground turkey or tofu provides a well-rounded, nutritious meal that supports blood sugar management, weight control, and overall health.

CHICKEN AND VEGETABLE CURRY WITH CAULIFLOWER RICE

Chicken and vegetable curry with cauliflower rice is a delicious and healthy option for individuals with prediabetes. This flavorful dish offers a wide range of benefits, both in terms of taste and nutrition.

The chicken in this curry provides a lean source of protein, which is important for individuals with prediabetes. Protein helps to stabilize blood sugar levels and can prevent post-meal spikes that are often associated with this condition. Additionally, chicken is low in fat, making it a heart-healthy choice.

The vegetables included in this curry are not only packed with essential nutrients, but they also add a burst of color and flavor to the dish. Vegetables such as bell peppers, carrots, and spinach are rich in vitamins, minerals, and antioxidants, which can help protect against chronic diseases like diabetes. These vegetables are also low in calories and high in fiber, promoting satiety and aiding in weight management – a crucial aspect of prediabetes management.

One of the highlights of this dish is the cauliflower rice. It is a clever low-carb alternative to traditional rice that makes it suitable for individuals with prediabetes. Cauliflower is an excellent source of fiber, vitamins C and K, and antioxidants. Its mild flavor and rice-like texture make it a perfect accompaniment to the flavorsome curry.

Preparing this dish is simple and requires a few steps. Start by cooking the chicken until it is tender and cooked through. In a separate pan, sauté the vegetables with fragrant spices like turmeric, cumin, and coriander. Once softened, add the chicken and a can of diced tomatoes. Simmer the mixture until the flavors meld together. While the curry is simmering, use a food processor to pulse the cauliflower florets into rice-like grains. Steam or sauté the cauliflower rice until it reaches the desired tenderness, and season it with salt and pepper to taste. Serve the chicken and vegetable curry over the cauliflower rice, and garnish with fresh cilantro for added flavor and visual appeal.

This chicken and vegetable curry with cauliflower rice is a nutritious and flavorful option for individuals with prediabetes. It offers a balanced combination of lean protein, vegetables, and a low-carb base, making it an ideal choice for those striving to manage blood sugar levels effectively.

BAKED COD WITH QUINOA AND SAUTÉED SPINACH

Baked cod with quinoa and sautéed spinach is an ideal meal for individuals with prediabetes, combining lean protein, fiber, and essential nutrients in a delicious and healthful dish. Each component of this meal offers specific benefits that contribute to blood sugar regulation and overall well-being.

Firstly, cod is a lean, low-calorie fish that provides high-quality protein, which is crucial for individuals with prediabetes. Protein helps to stabilize blood sugar levels by slowing the absorption of glucose into the bloodstream, preventing post-meal spikes that are often problematic for people with prediabetes. Additionally, protein promotes satiety, reducing hunger pangs and the likelihood of overeating, which can help in managing weight—a key factor in controlling prediabetes. Cod is also rich in omega-3 fatty acids, which have been shown to reduce inflammation and lower the risk of heart disease, a common complication in individuals with prediabetes. Omega-3 fatty acids are essential for cardiovascular health, supporting the heart and circulatory system in maintaining proper function.

Quinoa, a gluten-free whole grain, complements the cod perfectly by adding fiber, protein, and essential nutrients to the meal. The fiber content in quinoa is particularly beneficial for managing blood sugar levels. Fiber slows down the digestion process, resulting in a gradual release of glucose into the bloodstream, thus preventing rapid spikes in blood sugar levels. Quinoa is also considered a low-glycemic index food, meaning it has a minimal impact on blood sugar levels. This characteristic makes quinoa an excellent choice for individuals with prediabetes, as it promotes stable blood sugar control and reduces the risk of developing type 2 diabetes. Furthermore, quinoa is rich in magnesium, a mineral that plays a critical role in insulin sensitivity. Adequate magnesium intake can help improve the body's response to insulin, thereby aiding in blood sugar regulation.

Sautéed spinach adds a vibrant and nutritious element to the dish. Spinach is a nutrient powerhouse, rich in vitamins A, C, and K, as well as minerals like iron and magnesium. These vitamins and minerals are essential for overall health and can contribute to improved blood sugar management. For instance, vitamin A is important for maintaining healthy vision and immune function, vitamin C is a powerful antioxidant that helps protect cells from damage, and vitamin K plays a crucial role in blood clotting and bone health. Iron is necessary for the production of hemoglobin, which carries oxygen in the blood, and magnesium supports various biochemical reactions in the body, including those involved in blood sugar control. Spinach is also low in calories and carbohydrates, making it an excellent choice for individuals with prediabetes. The high fiber content in spinach can aid in maintaining healthy blood sugar levels by slowing digestion and promoting a feeling of fullness, which can help with weight management.

To prepare this nutritious and flavorful meal, start by seasoning the cod fillets with salt, pepper, and your choice of herbs or spices. Place the seasoned fish in a baking dish and bake it in the oven at 400°F (200°C) until it becomes tender and flaky, usually about 15-20 minutes. Meanwhile, cook the quinoa according to package instructions, using chicken or vegetable broth for added flavor. In a separate pan, heat olive oil and sauté the spinach until wilted, which typically takes about 3-5 minutes. Once everything is cooked, serve the baked cod on a bed of quinoa and top it with the sautéed spinach.

Baked cod with quinoa and sautéed spinach is a nutritious and delicious meal that provides numerous benefits for individuals with prediabetes. The combination of lean protein, low-glycemic index carbohydrates, and fiber-rich vegetables helps regulate blood sugar levels, reduce inflammation, and support overall health. By incorporating such balanced meals into their diet, individuals with prediabetes can effectively manage their condition and improve their quality of life.

TUNA SALAD ON WHOLE GRAIN BREAD WITH A SIDE OF RAW VEGGIES

Tuna salad on whole grain bread with a side of raw veggies is a delicious and nutritious meal suitable for individuals with prediabetes. Whole grain bread provides dietary fiber, aiding digestion and stabilizing blood sugar levels. It also contains essential nutrients like vitamins, minerals, and antioxidants. Tuna salad, made with lean tuna, is rich in protein and omega-3 fatty acids, which improve heart health, reduce inflammation, and enhance insulin sensitivity. This protein helps regulate blood sugar, preventing spikes and crashes.

Raw veggies such as carrots, cucumbers, and bell peppers add vital nutrients and fiber. These vegetables are rich in vitamins, minerals, and antioxidants, supporting overall health and reducing the risk of chronic diseases associated with prediabetes. The fiber in raw vegetables slows the absorption of sugar into the bloodstream, aiding glucose control.

To prepare this meal, make the tuna salad by mixing drained and flaked canned tuna with Greek yogurt, diced celery, chopped red onion, lemon juice, and seasonings. Lightly toast a slice of whole grain bread and spread the tuna salad evenly on it. Serve the sandwich with a side of washed and sliced raw veggies like carrot sticks, cucumber slices, and bell pepper strips. This meal combines the benefits of whole grain bread, lean protein from tuna, and nutrient-rich raw vegetables, creating a balanced and diabetes-friendly plate that supports blood sugar management and overall health.

GRILLED VEGETABLE WRAP WITH HUMMUS AND AVOCADO

The grilled vegetable wrap with hummus and avocado is a delicious and nutritious option for individuals with prediabetes. This wrap not only offers a burst of flavors but also provides numerous health benefits. The combination of grilled vegetables, hummus, and avocado ensures a filling and satisfying meal that helps maintain stable blood sugar levels.

Grilled vegetables are low in calories and high in fiber, making them ideal for those with prediabetes. Vegetables such as bell peppers, zucchini, and eggplant are packed with essential vitamins and minerals that support overall health. Grilling the vegetables enhances their natural flavors and adds a smoky taste, making them even more enjoyable.

Hummus, a popular Middle Eastern dip made from chickpeas, is a fantastic addition to this wrap. Chickpeas are high in fiber and have a low glycemic index, which means they release sugar into the bloodstream slowly, preventing spikes in blood sugar levels. Additionally, hummus is a good source of plant-based protein, making it an excellent substitute for high-glycemic ingredients like processed meats or cheese.

Avocado is another star ingredient in this recipe, known for its health-promoting properties. Rich in healthy fats, avocados can help improve insulin sensitivity and maintain a stable blood sugar level.

They are also loaded with fiber and essential nutrients like potassium and folate, which contribute to heart health and overall well-being.

To prepare this delicious wrap, start by grilling the vegetables until they become tender and slightly charred. Then, spread a generous amount of hummus over a whole wheat or low-carb tortilla. Next, layer the grilled vegetables on top of the hummus and add slices of ripe avocado. You can also include some fresh spinach or other leafy greens for added nutritional value. Finally, roll up the tortilla tightly and secure it with a toothpick or wrap it in parchment paper for easy handling.

This grilled vegetable wrap with hummus and avocado provides a balanced combination of vegetables, healthy fats, protein, and fiber, all of which contribute to stabilizing blood sugar levels and promoting overall health. By incorporating this delicious and nutritious wrap into their diet, individuals with prediabetes can enjoy a flavorful meal that supports their wellness goals.

LENTIL SOUP WITH A SIDE OF WHOLE GRAIN BREAD

Lentil soup with a side of whole grain bread is a wholesome and nourishing meal option for individuals with prediabetes. Lentils, a legume rich in protein and fiber, are the main ingredient in this soup, providing numerous health benefits. The low glycemic index of lentils helps regulate blood sugar levels, making them an excellent choice for prediabetic individuals. Additionally, lentils are packed with essential nutrients such as iron, magnesium, and folate, which play a crucial role in overall health and well-being.

The accompanying whole grain bread provides complex carbohydrates, which are beneficial in managing prediabetes. Unlike refined grains, whole grains are rich in fiber, offering a slow and steady release of glucose into the bloodstream, preventing blood sugar spikes. The fiber in whole grain bread also aids in digestion and helps maintain a healthy weight, which is crucial for prediabetic individuals. Moreover, whole grain bread is a good source of vitamins and minerals that support a balanced diet.

Preparing lentil soup with a side of whole grain bread is relatively simple. To begin, thoroughly rinse and drain the lentils before cooking. In a large pot, sauté onions, garlic, and other desired vegetables such as carrots and celery in a small amount of olive oil until they are tender. Add the lentils and vegetable broth to the pot, along with desired spices such as cumin, paprika, and thyme. Bring the mixture to a boil, then reduce the heat and let it simmer until the lentils are cooked and tender, usually around 25-30 minutes. Season with salt and pepper to taste.

Alongside the soup, whole grain bread can be toasted or served as is. To ensure the bread is truly whole grain, check the label for words like "whole wheat" or "whole grain" as the first ingredient. Whole grain bread can be enjoyed sliced and topped with a healthy spread such as hummus or avocado.

lentil soup with a side of whole grain bread into a prediabetic diet not only offers a satisfying and flavorsome meal but also promotes stable blood sugar levels. The combination of protein, fiber, and complex carbohydrates in this meal helps maintain a balanced diet while supporting optimal health for individuals with prediabetes.

QUINOA SALAD WITH MIXED VEGETABLES AND GRILLED SHRIMP

Quinoa salad with mixed vegetables and grilled shrimp is a delicious and nutritious dish that is perfect for individuals with prediabetes. This recipe combines the health benefits of quinoa, an ancient grain, with an array of colorful vegetables and lean protein. Quinoa is a great choice for prediabetes as it has a low glycemic index, meaning it does not cause a sharp rise in blood sugar levels. It is also high in fiber, protein, and essential nutrients such as magnesium, zinc, and iron, all of which are important for maintaining optimal health.

The preparation of this salad is straightforward. Begin by cooking the quinoa according to the package instructions and let it cool. Meanwhile, prepare the mixed vegetables by chopping a variety of vibrant vegetables like bell peppers, cherry tomatoes, cucumbers, and red onions. These vegetables are rich in vitamins, minerals, and antioxidants that can help reduce the risk of chronic diseases associated with prediabetes. Once the quinoa has cooled, toss it together with the mixed vegetables in a large bowl.

For the grilled shrimp, marinate them in a mixture of olive oil, garlic, lemon juice, and a pinch of salt and pepper for added flavor. Grill the shrimp for a few minutes on each side until they turn pink and opaque. Shrimp is a lean source of protein that contains omega-3 fatty acids, which have been shown to improve insulin sensitivity and reduce inflammation associated with prediabetes.

To assemble the salad, add the grilled shrimp on top of the quinoa and vegetable mixture. Drizzle a homemade dressing made from olive oil, lemon juice, minced garlic, and herbs like parsley and basil. This light and tangy dressing adds a refreshing taste to the salad without adding excessive calories or sugar.

VEGETABLE STIR-FRY WITH TOFU OR LEAN BEEF

Vegetable stir-fry with tofu or lean beef is a delicious and nutritious meal option that can be highly beneficial for individuals with prediabetes. Packed with an array of colorful vegetables and protein-rich tofu or lean beef, this dish provides a satisfying and balanced meal that can help stabilize blood sugar levels and support overall health.

The benefits of this dish lie in its low glycemic index, meaning it causes a slower and more gradual increase in blood sugar levels compared to high glycemic index foods. Including a variety of vegetables such as bell peppers, broccoli, carrots, and snow peas ensures an intake of essential vitamins, minerals, and dietary fiber. These nutrients help enhance insulin sensitivity, improve blood sugar control, and lower the risk of chronic conditions associated with prediabetes, such as heart disease and obesity.

Preparing vegetable stir-fry with tofu or lean beef is straightforward and can be tailored to personal preferences. Start by cutting the vegetables into bite-sized pieces and the tofu or lean beef into thin strips. In a heated non-stick pan or wok, add a small amount of heart-healthy oil, such as olive oil or sesame oil. Add garlic and ginger for extra flavor and sauté for a minute. Then, add the tofu or lean beef and cook until browned. Next, toss in the vegetables and stir-fry until they become tender yet still slightly crisp. Season with low-sodium soy sauce, a sprinkle of sesame seeds, or a drizzle of honey to enhance the flavors. Serve it over a bed of cooked brown rice or whole grain noodles for a satisfying and balanced meal.

BAKED CHICKEN WITH BROWN RICE AND ROASTED ASPARAGUS

Baked chicken with brown rice and roasted asparagus is a delicious and nutritious meal, especially beneficial for individuals with prediabetes. This dish combines lean protein, whole grains, and fiber-rich vegetables, helping to regulate blood sugar levels effectively.

Baked chicken serves as an excellent source of lean protein, essential for maintaining and repairing body tissues. Protein also keeps you feeling full longer, preventing overeating and helping stabilize blood sugar levels by slowing down glucose release. Baking the chicken instead of frying reduces unhealthy fat and calorie intake.

Brown rice is a healthier alternative to white rice due to its higher fiber content. Fiber helps control blood sugar by slowing glucose absorption, promoting digestive health, and reducing heart disease risk. Brown rice is also packed with vitamins, minerals, and antioxidants.

Roasted asparagus adds numerous health benefits. It is low in calories and rich in vitamins A, C, and K, as well as folate and potassium, which support cardiovascular health and blood pressure regulation. Asparagus contains the antioxidant glutathione, which prevents cellular damage and reduces inflammation, and its fiber content aids digestion and blood sugar regulation.

To prepare, marinate the chicken with herbs, spices, and olive oil, then bake until tender. Cook the brown rice according to package instructions. Trim and season the asparagus with olive oil, salt, and pepper, then roast until crisp. Serve the baked chicken over brown rice with a side of roasted asparagus for a balanced meal that supports healthy blood sugar management.

BAKED SALMON WITH QUINOA AND ROASTED BRUSSELS SPROUTS

Baked salmon with quinoa and roasted Brussels sprouts is a delicious and wholesome meal that offers numerous benefits for individuals with prediabetes. Salmon, the star of this dish, is an excellent source of high-quality protein and omega-3 fatty acids, which promote heart health and reduce inflammation—both crucial factors in managing prediabetes. Quinoa, a gluten-free grain, provides complex carbohydrates and fiber, aiding in blood sugar regulation and helping control post-meal glucose levels. Additionally, quinoa contains essential minerals such as magnesium and potassium, which support the body's overall metabolic functions. Roasted Brussels sprouts offer plenty of dietary fiber, vitamins, and antioxidants, contributing to better blood sugar control and reducing the risk of heart disease.

To prepare, marinate the salmon fillets in a mixture of lemon juice, garlic, and herbs, then bake until they reach a flaky texture. Season Brussels sprouts with olive oil, salt, and pepper, then roast until crispy. Cook quinoa separately and serve as a base for the baked salmon and roasted Brussels sprouts, creating a well-balanced and flavorful combination. This wholesome meal not only promotes stable blood sugar levels but also satisfies taste buds, making it an excellent choice for individuals with prediabetes.

TURKEY CHILI WITH MIXED BEANS AND VEGETABLES

Turkey chili with mixed beans and vegetables is a delicious and nutritious dish suitable for individuals with prediabetes. This hearty meal satisfies taste buds and offers numerous health benefits. Packed with protein from lean turkey, fiber from mixed beans, and an array of vitamins and minerals from various vegetables, this chili is ideal for maintaining stable blood sugar levels.

Turkey, as a lean source of protein, provides essential amino acids without excessive saturated fats, crucial for prediabetic individuals. Mixed beans, such as kidney beans, black beans, and chickpeas, are loaded with fiber that aids in slow digestion, preventing sudden spikes in blood sugar levels. The vegetable medley, including bell peppers, onions, tomatoes, zucchini, carrots, and corn, adds flavor and essential nutrients. These vegetables are rich in vitamins A and C, antioxidants, and dietary fiber, contributing to better overall health and blood sugar control.

The preparation of turkey chili with mixed beans and vegetables is simple. Start by browning ground turkey in a large pot or skillet using non-stick cooking spray to minimize added fats. Once the turkey is cooked, add finely chopped onions, bell peppers, and minced garlic. Sauté until the vegetables become tender and fragrant. Next, add canned mixed beans, preferably rinsed to reduce sodium content, along with canned diced tomatoes. For additional spice and flavor, incorporate chili powder, cumin, paprika, and a pinch of cayenne pepper. Allow the mixture to simmer over medium heat for 20-30 minutes to meld the flavors together.

The result is a hearty and flavorful turkey chili, packed with various vegetables and beans, perfect for individuals with prediabetes looking to improve their overall health and maintain stable blood sugar levels. This wholesome meal can be enjoyed alone or served with brown rice or whole-grain bread for added fiber and sustained energy. Regular consumption of this balanced dish can contribute to improved blood sugar management, weight control, and overall well-being.

GRILLED STEAK WITH A SIDE SALAD AND ROASTED SWEET POTATOES

Grilled steak with a side salad and roasted sweet potatoes is a delicious and nutritious meal suitable for individuals with prediabetes. This well-balanced dish offers numerous benefits for managing blood sugar levels and improving overall health.

Starting with the grilled steak, it provides a good source of protein, which helps stabilize blood sugar levels and promotes satiety. Protein takes longer to digest, preventing quick spikes in blood glucose levels. It also aids in building and repairing tissues, supporting muscle strength and growth. Opting for lean cuts of steak, such as sirloin or tenderloin, ensures a lower intake of saturated fat, reducing the risk of heart disease, a common concern for those with prediabetes.

The side salad adds an array of vitamins, minerals, and fiber. Leafy greens like spinach, kale, or romaine lettuce are high in nutrients and low in calories, aiding weight management, another important aspect of prediabetes management. Fiber-rich vegetables, such as cucumbers, bell peppers, and tomatoes, contribute to better blood glucose control by slowing down the absorption of carbohydrates. Additionally, the salad can be topped with healthy fats like avocado or nuts, which aid in better nutrient absorption and improve insulin sensitivity.

Roasted sweet potatoes offer an excellent alternative to starchy sides like white rice or mashed potatoes. Sweet potatoes have a lower glycemic index, meaning they cause a slower rise in blood sugar levels compared to high-glycemic foods. They are also rich in fiber, vitamins A and C, potassium, and antioxidants, all of which contribute to improved blood sugar regulation and overall well-being.

Preparing this dish is relatively simple. Season the steak with desired spices and grill it to your preferred level of doneness. Meanwhile, toss together a variety of fresh vegetables and leafy greens to create a colorful and nutritious side salad. Finally, coat sweet potato chunks with a small amount of olive oil, sprinkle with seasoning, and roast them in the oven until tender and slightly caramelized.

LEMON GARLIC SHRIMP WITH WHOLE WHEAT PASTA AND STEAMED BROCCOLI

Lemon garlic shrimp with whole wheat pasta and steamed broccoli is a tasty and nutritious meal ideal for individuals with prediabetes. Shrimp provides lean protein, crucial for stabilizing blood sugar levels and offering sustained energy, while its low saturated fat content supports heart health. The lemon and garlic add flavor without extra sodium or sugar, making it a great choice for managing prediabetes. Whole wheat pasta, a complex carbohydrate, digests slowly to prevent blood sugar spikes and is rich in fiber, aiding digestion and satiety. Steamed broccoli adds essential vitamins like C and K, as well as fiber, which helps regulate blood sugar. To prepare, sauté shrimp in olive oil with garlic and lemon juice, then combine with cooked whole wheat pasta and steamed broccoli, tossing everything together. This balanced meal provides lean protein, whole grains, and fiber-rich vegetables, making it an excellent option for blood sugar control and overall well-being.

FOOD LIST DICTIONARY

Apples

- Apples are relatively high in natural sugars, with about 19 grams of sugar in a medium-sized apple. Most of this sugar is fructose, which is a natural sugar found in fruits.

Artichokes

- Artichokes have a low sugar content, with less than 1 gram of sugar per medium artichoke. They are high in fiber and beneficial for digestion.

Asparagus

- Asparagus is very low in sugar, containing less than 2 grams of sugar per cup (about 134 grams). It's an excellent choice for a low-sugar vegetable.

Avocado

- Avocado has minimal sugar content, with about 0.2 grams of sugar per avocado. It is rich in healthy fats and fiber.

Bananas

- Bananas are relatively high in natural sugars, containing about 14 grams of sugar per medium-sized banana. The sugar content increases as the banana ripens.

Beets

- Beets have moderate sugar content, with about 9 grams of sugar per cup (about 136 grams) of cooked beets. They are rich in fiber and nutrients.

Bell Peppers

- Bell peppers have a low sugar content, with about 5 grams of sugar per cup (about 149 grams) of sliced bell peppers. Red bell peppers tend to be sweeter than green ones.

Blackberries

- Blackberries have relatively low sugar content compared to other fruits, with about 7 grams of sugar per cup (about 144 grams). They are high in fiber and antioxidants.

Blueberries

Blueberries have a moderate sugar content, with about 15 grams of sugar per cup (about 148 grams). They are packed with antioxidants and vitamins.

Broccoli

- Broccoli has very low sugar content, with about 2 grams of sugar per cup (about 91 grams) of chopped raw broccoli. It's high in fiber, vitamins, and minerals.

Brussels Sprouts

  - Brussels sprouts have low sugar content, with about 2 grams of sugar per cup (about 88 grams) of cooked Brussels sprouts. They are high in fiber, vitamins, and antioxidants.

Cabbage

- Cabbage has low sugar content, with about 3 grams of sugar per cup (about 89 grams) of chopped raw cabbage. It's a good source of fiber and vitamins.

Carrots

- Carrots contain moderate natural sugars, with about 5 grams of sugar per cup (about 128 grams) of chopped raw carrots. They are rich in beta-carotene and fiber.

Cauliflower

- Cauliflower has very low sugar content, with about 2 grams of sugar per cup (about 107 grams) of chopped raw cauliflower. It's high in fiber and vitamins.

Cherries

- Cherries are relatively high in natural sugars, with about 18 grams of sugar per cup (about 138 grams). They are also rich in antioxidants and vitamins.

Cranberries

   - Fresh cranberries have low sugar content, with about 4 grams of sugar per cup (about 100 grams). However, dried cranberries often have added sugars and can be much higher in sugar content.

Cucumbers

   - Cucumbers have very low sugar content, with about 2 grams of sugar per cup (about 104 grams) of sliced raw cucumber. They are mostly water and are low in calories.

Eggplant

   - Eggplant has low sugar content, with about 3 grams of sugar per cup (about 99 grams) of cooked eggplant. It's a good source of fiber and various nutrients.

Garlic

- Garlic has very low sugar content, with less than 1 gram of sugar per clove (about 3 grams). It's widely used for its flavor and potential health benefits.

Grapes

- Grapes are relatively high in natural sugars, with about 23 grams of sugar per cup (about 151 grams). They are also rich in vitamins and antioxidants.

Green Beans

- Green beans have low sugar content, with about 4 grams of sugar per cup (about 125 grams) of cooked green beans. They are also high in fiber and vitamins.

Kiwi

- Kiwi is relatively high in natural sugars, with about 13 grams of sugar per cup (about 180 grams) of sliced kiwi. They are rich in vitamin C and fiber.

Lettuce

- Lettuce has very low sugar content, with less than 1 gram of sugar per cup (about 36 grams) of shredded lettuce. It is also low in calories and provides vitamins and minerals.

Mango

- Mango is high in natural sugars, with about 46 grams of sugar per cup (about 165 grams) of sliced mango. It is also rich in vitamins A and C, and fiber.

Onions

- Onions have moderate sugar content, with about 9 grams of sugar per cup (about 160 grams) of chopped onions. They are also a good source of antioxidants and vitamins.

Oranges

- Oranges have moderate sugar content, with about 12 grams of sugar per medium orange (about 131 grams). They are an excellent source of vitamin C and fiber.

Papaya

- Papaya is relatively high in natural sugars, with about 11 grams of sugar per cup (about 145 grams) of sliced papaya. It is also rich in vitamins A and C, and fiber.

Peaches

- Peaches have moderate sugar content, with about 13 grams of sugar per medium peach (about 150 grams). They are also rich in vitamins A and C, and fiber.

Pineapple

   - Pineapple is high in natural sugars, with about
16 grams of sugar per cup (about 165 grams) of
pineapple chunks. It is also a good source of
vitamin C and bromelain, an enzyme that may help
digestion.

Plums

   - Plums have moderate sugar content, with
about 16 grams of sugar per cup (about 165 grams)
of sliced plums. They are also a good source of
vitamins A and C, and fiber.

Potatoes

   - Potatoes have low natural sugar content, with
about 2 grams of sugar per medium potato (about
213 grams). They are a good source of
carbohydrates, fiber, and vitamins like vitamin C
and B6.

Pumpkin

  - Pumpkin has low sugar content, with about 3 grams of sugar per cup (about 245 grams) of cooked, mashed pumpkin. It is also rich in vitamins A, C, and fiber.

Radishes

  - Radishes have very low sugar content, with less than 1 gram of sugar per cup (about 116 grams) of sliced radishes. They are also low in calories and provide vitamin C and potassium.

Raspberries

  - Raspberries have relatively low sugar content for fruits, with about 5 grams of sugar per cup (about 123 grams). They are high in fiber, vitamins C and K, and antioxidants.

Spinach

  - Spinach has very low sugar content, with less than 1 gram of sugar per cup (about 30 grams) of raw spinach. It is rich in vitamins A, C, K, and folate, as well as iron and calcium.

Strawberries

   - Strawberries have moderate sugar content, with about 7 grams of sugar per cup (about 152 grams) of sliced strawberries. They are also rich in vitamin C, manganese, and fiber.

Sweet Corn

   - Sweet corn has moderate sugar content, with about 6 grams of sugar per cup (about 164 grams) of cooked corn. It is also a good source of fiber, vitamins, and minerals.

Tomatoes

   - Tomatoes have low sugar content, with about 4 grams of sugar per medium tomato (about 123 grams). They are rich in vitamins A and C, potassium, and antioxidants like lycopene.

Watermelon

- Watermelon is relatively high in natural sugars, with about 9 grams of sugar per cup (about 152 grams) of diced watermelon. It is also high in vitamins A and C, and provides hydration due to its high water content.

Zucchini

- Zucchini has very low sugar content, with about 3 grams of sugar per medium zucchini (about 196 grams). It is low in calories and rich in vitamins A and C, as well as fiber.

FOODS TO AVOID FOR PREDIABETES AND THEIR SUBSTITUTES

1. Refined Grains

   - Avoid: White bread, white rice, regular pasta

   - Substitutes: Whole grain bread, brown rice, whole wheat pasta, quinoa

2. Sugary Beverages

   - Avoid: Soda, sweetened coffee and tea, energy drinks

   - Substitutes: Water, herbal tea, black coffee, unsweetened iced tea, sparkling water with a splash of lemon or lime

3. Sugary Snacks

   - Avoid: Candy, cookies, cakes, pastries

   - Substitutes: Fresh fruit, nuts, seeds, dark chocolate (in moderation), homemade baked goods with reduced sugar

4. Processed Foods

  - Avoid: Packaged snacks, ready-to-eat meals, processed meats

  - Substitutes: Homemade meals, fresh vegetables, lean meats, and homemade snacks

5. High Glycemic Index Vegetables

  - Avoid: Potatoes, corn

  - Substitutes: Sweet potatoes, carrots, cauliflower, leafy greens, zucchini

6. High-Fat Dairy Products

  - Avoid: Whole milk, full-fat cheese, cream

  - Substitutes: Skim milk, low-fat cheese, Greek yogurt, plant-based milk (unsweetened)

7. Fried Foods

  - Avoid: French fries, fried chicken, doughnuts

- Substitutes: Baked potatoes, grilled or baked chicken, air-fried or baked alternatives

8. High-Sugar Fruits

   - Avoid: Pineapple, watermelon, dried fruits

   - Substitutes: Berries, apples, pears, citrus fruits, fresh fruit in moderation

9. High-Sodium Foods

   - Avoid: Canned soups, salty snacks, processed meats

   - Substitutes: Low-sodium soups, unsalted nuts, fresh lean meats, herbs, and spices for seasoning

10. Sweetened Breakfast Cereals

   - Avoid: Sugary cereals, granola bars

   - Substitutes: Oatmeal, whole grain cereals, homemade granola, Greek yogurt with nuts and seeds

11. High-Sugar Desserts

   - Avoid: Ice cream, pudding, sweet pies

   - Substitutes: Frozen yogurt (no added sugar), chia seed pudding, fruit salad

12. Trans Fats

   - Avoid: Margarine, store-bought baked goods, fried fast foods

   - Substitutes: Olive oil, avocado oil, homemade baked goods, baked or grilled alternatives

13. Fruit Juices

   - Avoid: Orange juice, apple juice, grape juice (store-bought with added sugars)

   - Substitutes: Freshly squeezed juices in moderation, water with fruit slices, vegetable juices

14. Condiments with Added Sugar

- Avoid: Ketchup, barbecue sauce, salad dressings

- Substitutes: Homemade ketchup, mustard, salsa, vinaigrettes made with olive oil and vinegar

15. Alcoholic Beverages

- Avoid: Beer, sweet wines, cocktails with sugary mixers

- Substitutes: Dry wine, spirits with soda water, non-alcoholic beverages like kombucha

16. Sweetened Dairy Products

- Avoid: Flavored yogurt, sweetened milk drinks

- Substitutes: Plain Greek yogurt, unsweetened almond milk, add fresh fruit for flavor

17. Instant Oatmeal

- Avoid: Flavored instant oatmeal packets

- Substitutes: Steel-cut oats, rolled oats, add nuts and berries for sweetness

18. Canned Fruits in Syrup

   - Avoid: Fruit cocktails, canned fruits in heavy syrup

   - Substitutes: Fresh fruit, canned fruit in water or natural juice

19. High-Calorie Coffee Drinks

   - Avoid: Frappuccinos, lattes with flavored syrups

   - Substitutes: Black coffee, coffee with a splash of milk, homemade flavored coffee with cinnamon or vanilla extract

20. High-Sugar Breakfast Bars

   - Avoid: Commercial granola bars, breakfast pastries

   - Substitutes: Homemade granola bars with oats and nuts, whole fruit, a handful of nuts

21. White Flour Products

   - Avoid: White flour tortillas, white flour-based pastries

   - Substitutes: Whole wheat tortillas, almond flour or coconut flour-based baked goods

22. Sugary Sauces and Marinades

   - Avoid: Teriyaki sauce, sweet and sour sauce

   - Substitutes: Soy sauce with fresh ginger and garlic, homemade marinades using lemon juice, herbs, and spices

23. Breakfast Muffins

   - Avoid: Store-bought muffins, especially large ones

   - Substitutes: Homemade muffins with whole grains and reduced sugar, protein-packed egg muffins

24. Sweetened Condensed Milk

   - Avoid: Sweetened condensed milk in desserts and coffee

   - Substitutes: Evaporated milk, unsweetened almond milk with a bit of stevia

25. Sugary Energy Bars

   - Avoid: High-sugar energy bars

   - Substitutes: Nut and seed bars, homemade energy balls with dates and nuts

26. Sugary Spreads

   - Avoid: Jelly, jam, chocolate spreads

   - Substitutes: Nut butters, fresh fruit slices, mashed avocado

27. Instant Noodles

   - Avoid: Ramen, cup noodles with high sodium and carbs

- Substitutes: Whole grain noodles, spiralized vegetables, soba noodles

28. Processed Meat Products

   - Avoid: Sausages, bacon, hot dogs

   - Substitutes: Lean cuts of turkey or chicken, homemade meat patties with lean ground beef or turkey

29. Sweetened Nut Milks

   - Avoid: Sweetened almond milk, sweetened coconut milk

   - Substitutes: Unsweetened almond milk, unsweetened coconut milk, add your own natural sweeteners if needed

30. Candy Bars

   - Avoid: Milk chocolate candy bars

   - Substitutes: Dark chocolate (70% cocoa or higher), nuts and dried fruit mix (in moderation)

A COMPREHENSIVE PRE-DIABETIC 2-WEEK MEAL PLAN:

WEEK 1:

Day 1:

Breakfast: Scrambled eggs with sautéed mushrooms and whole wheat toast

Lunch: Chicken and vegetable curry with cauliflower rice

Dinner: Grilled shrimp skewers with a side salad and whole grain couscous

Day 2:

Breakfast: Quinoa porridge with almond milk, cinnamon, and a sprinkle of berries

Lunch: Baked tofu with quinoa and steamed vegetables

Dinner: Grilled chicken breast with roasted Brussels sprouts and brown rice

Day 3:

Breakfast: Greek yogurt with sliced almonds and a drizzle of honey

Lunch: Hummus and veggie wrap with a side of raw veggies

Dinner: Turkey chili with mixed beans and vegetables

Day 4:

Breakfast: Green smoothie with kale, spinach, banana, and almond milk

Lunch: Lentil and vegetable salad with a side of whole grain bread

Dinner: Baked salmon with quinoa and steamed broccoli

Day 5:

Breakfast: Whole grain toast with avocado and tomato slices

Lunch: Vegetable stir-fry with tofu or lean beef

Dinner: Grilled steak with a side salad and roasted

sweet potatoes

Day 6:

Breakfast: Quinoa salad with mixed vegetables and grilled shrimp

Lunch: Lemon garlic shrimp with whole wheat pasta and steamed broccoli

Dinner: Baked chicken with brown rice and roasted asparagus

Day 7:

Breakfast: Vegetable omelet with a side of whole wheat toast

Lunch: Spinach and feta salad with grilled chicken or shrimp

Dinner: Quinoa-stuffed bell peppers with lean ground turkey or tofu

WEEK 2:

Day 8:

Breakfast: Spinach and feta omelet with whole wheat toast

Lunch: Greek salad with grilled chicken

Dinner: Grilled steak with a side salad and roasted sweet potatoes

Day 9:

Breakfast: Quinoa-stuffed bell peppers with lean ground turkey or tofu

Lunch: Turkey chili with mixed beans and vegetables

Dinner: Baked salmon with quinoa and roasted Brussels sprouts

Day 10:

Breakfast: Baked tofu with roasted sweet potatoes and steamed green beans

Lunch: Lemon garlic shrimp with whole wheat

pasta and steamed broccoli

Dinner: Grilled chicken breast with steamed vegetables

Day 11:

Breakfast: Quinoa salad with mixed vegetables and grilled shrimp

Lunch: Vegetable stir-fry with tofu or lean beef

Dinner: Baked chicken with brown rice and roasted asparagus

Day 12:

Breakfast: Oatmeal with berries and a sprinkle of nuts

Lunch: Lentil soup with a side of whole grain bread

Dinner: Grilled vegetable wrap with hummus and avocado

Day 13:

Breakfast: Yogurt with mixed berries and a sprinkle of chia seeds

Lunch: Tuna salad on whole grain bread with a side of raw veggies

Dinner: Greek salad with grilled chicken or shrimp

Day 14:

Breakfast: Veggie and bean burrito bowl with brown rice and salsa

Lunch: Black bean and vegetable enchiladas with a side of salsa and brown rice

Dinner: Baked cod with quinoa and sautéed spinach

CONCLUSION

In managing prediabetes, making informed dietary choices is essential to maintaining stable blood sugar levels and promoting overall health. This book, "The Prediabetes Food List," provides a comprehensive guide to understanding the nutritional value of various foods and their impact on blood sugar. By highlighting the importance of low glycemic index foods, fiber-rich vegetables, lean proteins, and whole grains, the book equips readers with practical knowledge to make healthier choices and support their journey towards better metabolic health.

The emphasis on whole, nutrient-dense foods helps to prevent sudden spikes in blood glucose levels while ensuring that your diet is both satisfying and balanced. By incorporating foods like quinoa, lean meats, and a variety of fruits and vegetables, individuals with prediabetes can enjoy meals that not only taste great but also contribute to their long-term health goals.

Understanding the sugar content and glycemic impact of different foods allows for better planning and more informed decision-making, making it easier to adhere to dietary recommendations. This book encourages a proactive approach to health, empowering readers to take control of their eating habits and ultimately improve their well-being.

Adopting the strategies and food choices outlined in The "Prediabetes Food List" can pave the way to effective prediabetes management. By focusing on nutrient-rich foods and maintaining a balanced diet, individuals can better manage their blood sugar levels, reduce the risk of progression to type 2 diabetes, and lead a healthier, more fulfilling life.

www.ingramcontent.com/pod-product-compliance
Lightning Source LLC
Chambersburg PA
CBHW071550260726
48653CB00007BA/2690